Mental Health Journal for Women

Mental Health Journal
for Women

Creative Prompts and Practices to Improve Your Well-Being

Sana Isaac Powell, MA, LPC

**ROCKRIDGE
PRESS**

For general information on our other products and services or to obtain technical support, please contact our Customer Care Department within the United States at (866) 744-2665, or outside the United States at (510) 253-0500.

Rockridge Press publishes its books in a variety of electronic and print formats. Some content that appears in print may not be available in electronic books, and vice versa.

Interior and Cover Designer: Jenny Paredes
Art Producer: Janice Ackerman
Editor: Eun H. Jeong
Production Editor: Ashley Polikoff

All illustrations used under license from iStock

Author Photo Courtesy of Zach Brigham Photography.

ISBN: 978-1-638-78881-2
R0

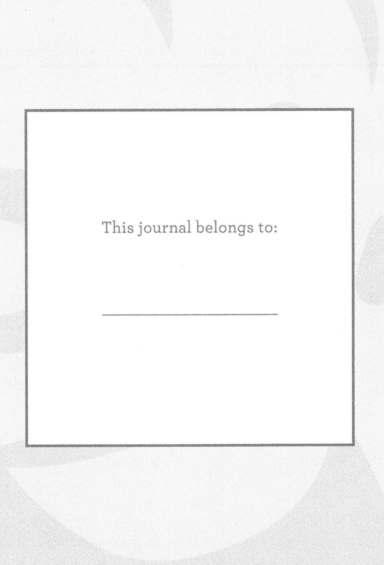

This journal belongs to:

_____

Contents

Introduction

Welcome to *Mental Health Journal for Women*, a supportive space for nurturing your psychological, emotional, and social well-being. My name is Sana Powell, and I'm a holistic and culturally affirming licensed professional counselor (LPC). I earned my BS in biopsychology, cognition, and neuroscience from the University of Michigan and my MA in mental health counseling and behavioral medicine from the Boston University School of Medicine. I have worked with diverse populations and treated issues ranging from generalized anxiety and depression to schizophrenia and severe substance use disorders.

Throughout my work, I've been drawn to the unique experiences of women and how their mental health is shaped by factors such as culture, personality, social environment, and biology.

According to the National Institute of Mental Health, some mental health issues are more prevalent in women than in men, such as anxiety and depression. Additionally, certain mental health disorders are specific to women and influenced by hormonal changes, like perinatal depression, premenstrual dysphoric disorder, and perimenopause-related depression.

It can be easy to ignore signs of declining mental health, such as chronic stress, irritability, trouble sleeping, and difficulty focusing—especially as feeling overworked is often glamorized by society. It is critical that women are equipped with tools to care for their own mental health. This journal will help boost your confidence in caring for yourself holistically, considering the connectedness between your mental, emotional, and physical well-being.

This book was largely influenced by my own experiences as a first-generation Indian-American woman. I have often felt lost at the intersection of my identities and thankfully have learned to navigate them by accepting and celebrating them. Whatever identities you may hold in addition to being a woman, I encourage you to embrace them as you move through this journal.

As you engage in this intimate inner work, take time to acknowledge if uncomfortable emotions or memories arise, and honor your limits. This book is not a replacement for therapy, so please seek out mental health treatment if you'd like individualized support in helping you cope with your thoughts and emotions. May this journal support you in your pursuit to improve your mental well-being as you make peace with your past, savor your present, and look ahead to your future.

How to Use
This Journal

Using this journal will help you reflect on, process, and externalize your inner experience in healthy ways. As mental health is multifaceted, so is this journal. It will allow you to explore your psychological, emotional, and social well-being: all essential aspects of mental health.

Part one will encourage you to tap into your emotions as you practice self-compassion and self-acceptance. Next, part two will help you master your mindset by developing thought patterns that are growth-oriented and sustainable. Lastly, part three will help you thrive in your social life, as you gain helpful communication tools and dismantle barriers to experiencing more fulfilling and meaningful relationships.

Throughout this journal, you will come across reflective writing prompts, creative exercises, mindful practices, and encouraging affirmations to help you nurture your mental well-being. The activities in this journal reflect concepts related to cognitive behavioral therapy (CBT), dialectical behavior therapy (DBT), mindfulness, positive psychology, and more. CBT focuses on identifying and changing unhelpful thought patterns that negatively impact your emotions and behaviors. DBT, a form of CBT, highlights developing healthy ways to cope with stress, manage your emotions, improve your relationships with others, and live in the moment, or be mindful. *Mindfulness* broadly describes the concept of being aware of, and compassionate toward, yourself and your experiences to achieve a greater sense of well-being in both mind and body. Lastly, positive psychology involves identifying and cultivating your strengths to lead a happier and more meaningful life. While the varied activities in each part of this journal work together to benefit your mental health, they also stand alone. You can move through this journal in a way that feels comfortable for you, whether you complete each activity sequentially or out of order.

As you progress through this journal, try sitting with your inner experience, resisting the urge to ignore, label, or judge it. Simply acknowledge and make space for thoughts and emotions. Remember that within moments of discomfort you may find glimmers of growth, insight, and healing. Challenge yourself to step out of your comfort zone and enjoy the process of getting to know yourself better. Your mental health is like a muscle that you can strengthen over time. Doing this inner work is no small feat, so acknowledge all your efforts and remember that cultivating mental health is a daily process. The more you give of yourself, the more you'll get in return.

Part
One

Tap Into Your Emotions

How often do you honestly answer the question, "How are you?" In the midst of our busy lives, it can be easy to go days, weeks, or even months without acknowledging—even to ourselves—how we truly feel. We may also avoid our emotions (either knowingly or unknowingly) by focusing on our achievements and the emotions of others. If the thought of tapping into your emotions feels awkward or intimidating, that's okay. Being vulnerable in this way can be challenging, and it's all right if you don't have much experience doing so. This part of the journal will help you nurture your emotional well-being with the help of reflective writing prompts, exercises, practices, and affirmations. You'll explore the topics of emotional awareness, stress management, self-expression, resiliency, and more.

    As you progress through this part of the journal, experiment with stepping out of what's comfortable and sitting with your emotions without judgment. Doing this reflective work to examine and understand the complexity of your emotions will help you connect with and manage them in a healthy way.

What you hold inside gets heavy over time. Write about things that have been weighing on you that you haven't had the chance to express. You deserve to be able to finally set down the heavy load you've been carrying.

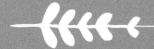

I am worthy. I am safe. I am cherished.
I will acknowledge my needs and
nourish my mind, body, and spirit.

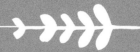

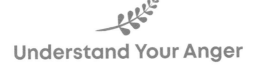

Understand Your Anger

Anger is a natural emotion that can offer valuable information about our needs and preferences. Sometimes anger may also hide underlying emotions that we're not comfortable expressing. Think of a time when you felt angry, and circle the emotions that you may have also felt at the time. Gently peel back the layers of your anger, and avoid judging or criticizing yourself through the process. This might feel difficult at first, but remind yourself that it gets easier with practice.

Disrespected	Disappointed	Violated	Frustrated
Vulnerable	Overwhelmed	Jealous	Humiliated
Ashamed	Uncomfortable	Guilty	Hurt
Threatened	Exhausted	Scared	Resentful
Annoyed	Abandoned	Embarrassed	Attacked
Betrayed	Sad	Dismissed	Insecure
Awkward	Bitter	Regretful	Trapped

Making space for your emotions can allow you to practice self-acceptance and better understand how you respond to the world around you. Exploring emotions without minimizing them cultivates vulnerability. This might feel difficult at first, but remind yourself that it gets easier with practice.

Write a letter to your younger self. Tell yourself what you needed to hear, give yourself the safety you might have craved, and comfort your inner child with what you know now. Write with compassion to that child still within you.

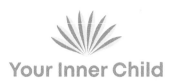

Your Inner Child

Reconnect with and nurture your inner child by doing something that brought you joy in your childhood. Perhaps it's having a good laugh with friends, dancing to your favorite song, going on a bike ride, or eating your favorite dessert before dinner. Whatever it may be, allow yourself the pleasure of doing something that gave you joy as a child. If you feel silly or awkward while doing it, you're likely on the right track! You may even find that incorporating playfulness into your life helps you cope with stress and produces a more positive outlook when dealing with difficult situations. It's important to acknowledge what emotions naturally come up for you as you reflect on your childhood. If reconnecting with your inner child makes you feel anxious or uncomfortable, that's okay. Honor your boundaries and remember that you can tap into your inner child whenever you feel ready.

Body neutrality is about accepting your body and appreciating its capabilities instead of focusing on, or solely loving it for, its appearance. Write three statements of gratitude for what your body can do that are independent of how it looks.

Thank you, body, for ....

....

....

....

Thank you, body, for ....

....

....

....

Thank you, body, for ....

....

....

....

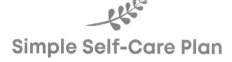

Simple Self-Care Plan

Burnout, or a state of emotional, physical, and mental exhaustion, results from stress that builds up over time. To help avoid burn-out, create a simple self-care plan that you can utilize. Focus on self-care ideas that you can easily do, such as deep breathing, taking a power nap, calling a friend, going for a walk, listening to music, journaling, or exercising. Choose self-care practices that align with your lifestyle and preferences.

When I feel overwhelmed, I will:

1. ....

2. ....

When I feel stressed, I will:

1. ....

2. ....

When I feel anxious, I will:

1. ....

2. ....

When I feel lonely, I will:

1. ....

2. ....

When I feel tired, I will:

1. ....

2. ....

When I feel irritable, I will:

1. ....

2. ....

The simpler a self-care practice is, the more likely you are to consistently use it. Check in with yourself periodically, and use your self-care plan to manage your stress levels and avoid burnout.

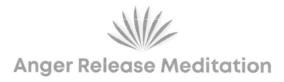

Anger Release Meditation

If you're not ready to fully let go of your anger, that's okay. Just allow yourself to loosen your grip on it.

1. Find a comfortable position and relax the muscles in your face. Drop your shoulders and soften your jaw.

2. Take slow, deep breaths as you breathe in through your nose and out through your mouth. Place a hand on your lower belly and feel it rise as you inhale.

3. Hold your breath for a moment at the top of each inhale before slowly releasing it. Notice how your muscles gradually soften with each exhale.

4. Repeat this practice 3 to 7 times.

Releasing your anger does not invalidate how you feel. Rather, it can allow you to address your emotions by practicing self-love. It can also help you adopt a new perspective and make space for more peace in your life.

What did this deep breathing meditation feel like for you? What did you learn about yourself? How does your body feel after the practice compared to before?

_____

_____

_____

_____

_____

_____

_____

_____

_____

_____

_____

_____

_____

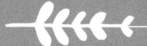

I am secure in myself, and I embrace
my flaws with self-compassion.
My imperfections make me strong,
unique, and beautiful.

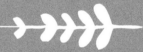

What are some things you do (or don't do) that hold you back from growth? Perhaps it's procrastination, lack of confidence, self-criticism, self-isolation, substance misuse, engaging in harmful behaviors, or something else. Without criticizing yourself, list five things that have been holding you back.

1. ....

....

2. ....

....

3. ....

....

4. ....

....

5. ....

....

Holistic Self-Care Assessment

Your inner child craves for your basic needs to be met. Take some time to reflect on self-care across different areas of your life, and circle the responses that fit best.

Psychological and Emotional:
I maintain a healthy mindset, make time for self-reflection, and allow myself to experience my emotions.

| Strongly Disagree | Disagree | Neutral | Agree | Strongly Agree |

Physical:
I take care of my body by staying hydrated, nourishing it with healthy foods, resting, and staying active within my limits.

| Strongly Disagree | Disagree | Neutral | Agree | Strongly Agree |

Social:
I have a reliable support system, I communicate my needs, and I set appropriate boundaries with others.

| Strongly Disagree | Disagree | Neutral | Agree | Strongly Agree |

Notice the areas of your life in which you circled "Strongly Disagree," "Disagree," or "Neutral," and consider if they could use some extra nurturing.

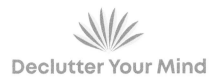

Declutter Your Mind

Practice self-love by tidying up your space. Whether you live in a cluttered space or not, challenge yourself to stretch from your comfort zone with this exercise. According to a 2009 study, a cluttered space can lead to stress, which can eventually lead to mental and physical health issues.

Choose a space in your home to declutter. If you feel overwhelmed, do as much as you comfortably can, and use this checklist as a guide:

- Take out the trash.
- Pick up dirty clothes.
- Donate things you don't use.
- Organize your belongings.
- Vacuum or sweep the floor.

The messier our living spaces are, the more challenging it can be to sift through them to find what we're looking for, create space for what we need, and do what we have planned. Part of removing barriers to our growth involves decluttering our lives and, consequently, our minds.

> *Mild anxiety can be helpful in motivating us to meet deadlines, alerting us that something is important to us, and protecting us from potential danger. Write about one or a few things that make you anxious and what your anxiety might be trying to tell you.*

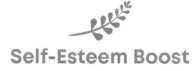

Self-Esteem Boost

Don't be shy! Take a moment to acknowledge your achievements, no matter how big or small.

If complimenting yourself feels difficult, consider what your friends would say they like about you.

I'm proud of myself for:

1. ....

2. ....

3. ....

Things I like about myself are:

1. ....

2. ....

3. ....

Write down a few of the biggest challenges you've faced, and remind yourself of how far you've already come.

In my life I've overcome:

1. ....

2. ....

3. ....

People say my strengths are:

1. ....

2. ....

3. ....

It's okay if you don't feel fully confident in yourself in this moment. Write your future achievements into existence anyway.

The goals I'll achieve are:

1. ....

2. ....

3. ....

I feel most confident when:

1. ....

2. ....

3. ....

We all have insecurities—they might be related to our abilities, physical appearance, background, or something else. Write about an insecurity you have and where it may stem from. As you reflect, remember to practice self-compassion and treat yourself the way you'd treat a dear friend.

_____

_____

_____

_____

_____

_____

_____

_____

_____

_____

_____

_____

_____

_____

_____

_____

_____

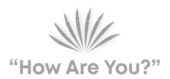

"How Are You?"

Let's circle back to something I asked at the beginning of this book: When was the last time you honestly answered the question, "How are you?" If you're like most people, you probably answer this question with automatic, general responses ("good," "fine," "okay") that may have nothing to do with how you're really feeling. This is normal—social pressure can make women feel like we always have to be positive, bubbly, or friendly, even if we feel otherwise.

The next time someone you care about asks how you're doing, challenge yourself to answer honestly. For example, mention something that you feel proud of yourself for achieving, something that you've felt stressed about, or a goal you've been working toward. Practice sharing your thoughts and emotions, and be open to the conversations that your honesty elicits. Being vulnerable in this way might feel intimidating at first because it risks experiencing rejection. Remember that, regardless of the outcome, you invest in your mental health when you practice vulnerability—and you are well worth the investment. Besides, they asked!

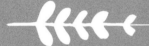

I have made it through 100 percent of my worst days, and I am strong enough to handle whatever comes my way.

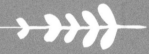

Recall a time when you were faced with a challenge you didn't think you could overcome, but you did. Consider the strength, courage, and perseverance it took for you to overcome this challenge and what reflecting on this memory feels like.

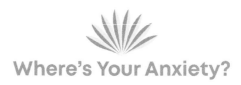

Where's Your Anxiety?

1. Find a comfortable position and take slow, deep breaths, breathing in through your nose and out through your mouth.

2. Now think of a person, place, or thing that makes you feel mildly anxious. Try to envision as many details as you can.

3. Notice what sensations arise in your body. Perhaps it's a racing heart, tightness in your chest, sweaty palms, shallow breathing, or tense muscles. Acknowledge how these sensations feel different from how your body felt before you began the practice.

4. After a few moments, bring your attention back to your breath and remind yourself that you are safe and in control.

Anxiety is related to the body's sympathetic nervous system, commonly known as your fight-or-flight response. When your mind perceives a threat, it signals your body to protect itself. Becoming aware of these physical sensations can help you better identify when you're beginning to feel anxious.

Reflect on your experience with this visualization exercise. What thoughts came up for you? What sensations did you feel in your body?

We can be so hard on ourselves sometimes, criticizing ourselves and focusing on our flaws. This is not surprising, given the influence of society's impossibly skewed standards for a woman's appearance, status, and achievements. Take a moment to list five things that make you feel confident about yourself. If this is challenging, think about how a loved one would describe you.

1. ....

....

2. ....

....

3. ....

....

4. ....

....

5. ....

....

When we're feeling overwhelmed, knowing how to calm ourselves is essential for our mental health. List five things that can help you feel more relaxed, grounded, and healthy in moments of stress (such as talking with friends, meditating, exercising, journaling, getting enough sleep, deep breathing, etc.).

1. ....

....

2. ....

....

3. ....

....

4. ....

....

5. ....

....

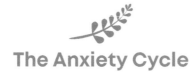

The Anxiety Cycle

Take a moment to identify something that makes you anxious (this is an "anxiety trigger") and what your experience is like when you avoid that trigger. Reflect on the questions below for each stage in the cycle of anxiety, beginning with your anxiety trigger.

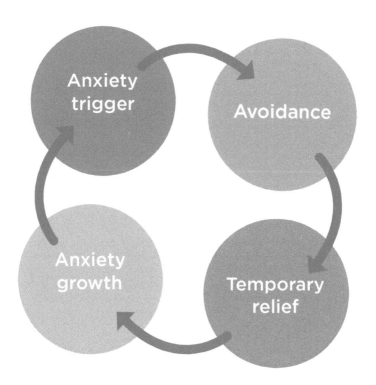

Anxiety trigger: What situation, person, place, or thing makes you feel significantly worried, fearful, or overwhelmed?

Avoidance: How do you avoid your anxiety? For example, some people might procrastinate or use substances to numb their emotions.

Temporary relief: How does avoiding your anxiety feel in the short-term?

Anxiety growth: Over time, unresolved anxiety might show up as a fast heart rate, chest tightness, or excessive sweating. What does worsening anxiety feel like for you?

While avoiding your anxiety may provide short-term relief, it can worsen your anxiety over time. The good news is that you can disrupt this cycle by identifying and coping with whatever's making you anxious. Seek support from a mental health professional if your anxiety feels uncontrollable or holds you back from living a fulfilling life.

When was the last time you felt burnt out mentally, emotionally, or physically? Looking back, what contributed to your exhaustion? What could you have done differently to prevent getting to the point of burnout?

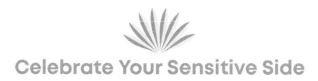

Celebrate Your Sensitive Side

Identify one thing that nudges you to embrace your vulnerability and acknowledge your true feelings. Perhaps it's engaging in an activity that feels therapeutic and helps you process your thoughts and emotions (listening to music, creating art, going on a walk, gardening, etc.). Maybe it's reaching out to a friend to check on them, share your feelings, or ask for support. It could even be allowing yourself to feel your emotions instead of ignoring them, even if that means allowing yourself to cry. Whatever it may be, take time to honor your identity as a sentient being who uniquely perceives and reacts to the world around you. If tapping into your sensitivity feels awkward or uncomfortable, that's okay. Avoid criticizing yourself for whatever emotions may surface, and remember that there's no "right" or "wrong" outcome from this practice. Be open to however it naturally unfolds.

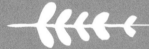

My worth is not defined by my appearance or weight. Who I am is so much more than my physical appearance.

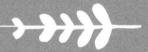

Today, reflect on something you lost that causes you some sadness. Perhaps it was the loss of a person, pet, relationship, or part of yourself that you never processed. This is your time to let it out without shame or judgment.

Sometimes we close ourselves off from emotional vulnerability after being hurt and miss out on the beauty of vulnerability with the right people. Reflect on how comfortable you are with being vulnerable and expressing your emotions. Consider how your past relationships and experiences might influence this.

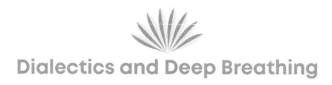

Dialectics and Deep Breathing

1. It's natural to grieve the loss of something even if you know it was unhealthy for you. Identify one unhealthy thing that's no longer a part of your life but that you still miss some-times (a harmful relationship, a toxic habit, an unhealthy lifestyle, etc.). Write it in the space below:

I can miss

AND

still know I made the right decision for my mental health.

_____

2. Now find a comfortable position and take slow, deep breaths, breathing in through your nose and out through your mouth.

3. Repeat the statement you created in step 1 out loud to yourself as you continue breathing. Close your eyes or lower your gaze if it helps you feel more grounded.

Dr. Marsha Linehan, psychologist and the creator of dialectical behavior therapy, describes this as a dialectical practice, or one that accommodates the truth of two contrasting ideas. Use this practice whenever you want to embrace both change and accep-tance as you cope with loss.

How did it feel holding space for two conflicting ideas? What emotions came up for you?

_____

_____

_____

_____

_____

_____

_____

_____

_____

_____

_____

_____

_____

Emotional sensitivity or vulnerability is often portrayed as weakness, when in reality, it is a tremendous strength. How comfortable are you with being sensitive and holding space for the sensitivity of others? What messages did you receive around sensitivity while growing up?

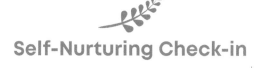

Self-Nurturing Check-in

Check in with yourself about how nurtured you feel today. Practice self-compassion through this check-in. Resist the urge to criticize or judge yourself based on your responses. There is no shame in growth.

	True	False	Unsure
I feel rested today.			
I allow myself to feel my emotions.			
I feel hydrated.			
My body feels nourished.			
I've moved my body in a healthy way today.			
My body feels relaxed.			
I feel grounded and at ease.			
I'm conscious of my screen time.			
I've set realistic goals for the day.			
I've genuinely smiled or laughed today.			
I've been practicing good personal hygiene.			

If you responded with "False" or "Unsure" to any of the questions above, it may indicate areas of potential growth for simple self-nurturing. Remember that self-nurturing is an individual process, and while this check-in can provide ideas on where to start, seek out self-nurturing practices that work for you and fit your unique lifestyle and preferences.

Self-nurturing involves a daily practice of caring for ourselves, practicing self-compassion, and acknowledging our needs. List five ways you will nurture yourself today (such as staying hydrated, moving your body, cooking your favorite meal, buying yourself flowers, reading a good book, etc.).

1. ....

....

2. ....

....

3. ....

....

4. ....

....

5. ....

....

When was the last time you felt angry? Where were you? Was anyone else with you? Take a few minutes to write about this memory as you reflect on the details of what happened and how it made you feel.

_____

_____

_____

_____

_____

_____

_____

_____

_____

_____

_____

_____

_____

_____

_____

_____

Helpful vs. Unhelpful Coping Skills

As humans, it's natural to cope with stress in whatever ways we can. Instead of labeling our coping skills based on how healthy they are, let's conceptualize them based on how *helpful* they are. Helpful coping skills benefit us in the short and long term, don't hurt ourselves or others, and are sustainable. Unhelpful coping skills provide temporary relief but cause hurt in the long term (substance misuse, engaging in harmful behaviors, self-criticism, etc.). List coping skills you've used in the past as well as helpful coping skills you'd like to try in the future:

Helpful Coping Skills	Unhelpful Coping Skills

Whether the ways you've coped with stress in the past were helpful or unhelpful, they've allowed you to be here today—and there is no shame in that. Be kind to yourself as you adopt more helpful and sustainable practices for coping with stress. This is a lifelong journey.

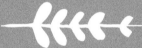

My feelings matter. I will acknowledge my emotions with love and acceptance and freely express myself in healthy ways.

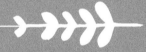

Part
Two

Master Your Mindset

Gaining insight into our psychological processes is a critical aspect of mental health. Many of the ways we react to ourselves and others are somewhat automatic, so recognizing the familiar patterns we've developed is the first step in disrupting harmful cycles and incorporating helpful practices. Part two of this journal will help you nurture your psychological well-being by increasing your self-awareness and then using that awareness to cultivate a mindset that is healthy, sustainable, and growth-oriented. Some topics you'll explore include gratitude, overthinking, decision-making, compassion, motivation, and more.

You'll be encouraged to recognize your core values, consider your self-beliefs, and identify any barriers to personal growth. As you progress through this section, you may feel challenged by activities that ask you to reflect on the past, accept the present, and look ahead to the future in ways that you haven't done before. If difficult thoughts or emotions arise, create a safe environment for yourself. You can do this by replacing self-criticism with self-compassion and reminding yourself that a little discomfort often accompanies growth. Acknowledge your efforts and remember that cultivating a healthy mindset is a daily process.

Self-forgiveness is about accepting the consequences of your actions, learning from them, and moving forward with intention. You deserve to experience the freedom and peace that self-forgiveness offers. What would you like to forgive yourself for?

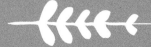

Any trauma I experienced was not
my fault. I hold space for it and know
that it does not define me.

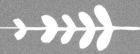

Instead of withholding love from yourself until you accomplish a goal or are somehow different from who you are today, practice radical self-acceptance. What parts of yourself can you offer some extra love and compassion?

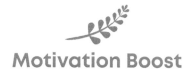

Motivation Boost

Telling yourself that you "should" do something you've been feeling unmotivated to do can minimize your emotions and sense of autonomy. Over time, this may lead to feelings of anxiety, dread, and even resentment. Examine your thoughts and emotions surrounding something you've been putting off.

Complete the following statement with something you think you should do that you've been feeling unmotivated about:

I really should ....

....

Acknowledge three barriers:

Some things that get in the way of doing this are:

1. ....

2. ....

3. ....

Focus on your values:

Doing this is important to me because ....

....

Consider the positive emotions that could come from it:

After I do this, I'll feel ....

....

Incorporate gratitude:

I'm thankful I get to do this because ....

....

When you find yourself using the word *should* related to some-thing you've been putting off, use this exercise to gain insight and feel more motivated, intentional, and empowered.

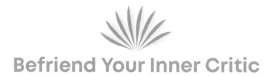

Befriend Your Inner Critic

Our inner critic refers to the inner voice that often judges or belittles us. It might tell you that you're not good enough, not smart enough, or not attractive enough. At the core, it might make you feel like you are inherently inadequate in some way. Over time, this can deteriorate your self-esteem and mental health. The next time you experience negative self-talk or self-critical thoughts, try to challenge these thoughts instead of immediately accepting them as truth. Consider what evidence supports your negative self-talk and what evidence affirms your capabilities.

Also, consider how your inner critic might be trying to protect you. Is it trying to shield you from pain, failure, or rejection? Acknowledging your inner critic and viewing it through a more compassionate lens can help you gradually replace negative self-talk with positive self-talk or affirming and uplifting thoughts about yourself.

Practicing gratitude doesn't minimize or dismiss the struggles you may be facing. Rather, it makes space for joy, even in the midst of adversity. List 10 things in your life that you're grateful for (people, pets, experiences, things, etc.).

1. ....

2. ....

3. ....

4. ....

5. ....

6. ....

7. ....

8. ....

9. ....

10. ....

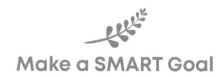

Make a SMART Goal

Falling short in achieving goals isn't a reflection of our capabilities but rather an indication that we can improve our goal-setting skills. SMART, an acronym developed by George Doran in 1981, can help with this:

Specific: What do you specifically want to accomplish?

Measurable: How will you determine whether you're making progress?

Achievable: Can you realistically accomplish the goal?

Relevant: Is the goal important to you, and does it align with your values?

Time-based: When will the goal be completed and evaluated?

Example of an unclear goal: "I'll do things to help decrease my anxiety."

Example of a SMART goal: "For two weeks, I will spend at least 15 minutes each day doing at least one relaxing activity (reading, meditation, listening to music, etc.) to help reduce the symptoms of my anxiety (racing thoughts, restlessness, tense muscles, etc.)."

Draft your SMART goal, making sure to focus on progress over perfection.

_____

_____

_____

_____

_____

_____

_____

_____

_____

_____

_____

_____

_____

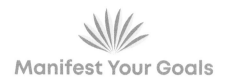

Manifest Your Goals

Visualizing success can help you build the self-confidence it takes to achieve it. Let's try it.

1. Find a comfortable position and relax the muscles in your face. Drop your shoulders and soften your jaw. Close your eyes or lower your gaze if it helps you feel less distracted.

2. Take slow, deep breaths, breathing in through your nose and out through your mouth. Place a hand on your lower belly and feel it rise as you inhale.

3. Hold your breath for a moment at the top of each inhale before slowly releasing it. Notice how your muscles gradually soften with each exhale.

4. As you breathe, imagine yourself achieving a goal you've been working toward. Visualize this successful outcome in your life, picturing as many details as you can.

5. Remind yourself that you are capable of achieving your goals.

6. Conclude this meditation whenever you feel ready to do so.

What goal did you visualize achieving, and why is achieving it important to you? What's one thing you can do today to move closer to this goal?

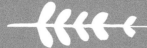

No matter how difficult or daunting a challenge may be, I will overcome it because I am capable, strong, and resilient.

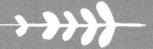

We are our own biggest critics. Write down three to five self-critical thoughts that have been negatively impacting your mental health. While this might feel uncomfortable at first, remember that letting thoughts out is often healthier than holding them in.

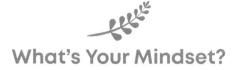

What's Your Mindset?

Choose the response that best describes your typical mindset, and accept yourself for who you are in this moment.

1. When I fail at something . . .
   A. It's a sign that I'm not capable.
   B. It's an opportunity for growth.
   C. I might give up on trying.

2. My skills and abilities . . .
   A. Are mostly unchangeable.
   B. Are influenced by my effort and attitude.
   C. Might grow a little over time.

3. When I receive constructive criticism . . .
   A. I get defensive or ignore it.
   B. I reflect on potential areas of growth.
   C. I might consider it.

Insights

◆ If you chose mostly As, you might have a fixed mindset. *Try experimenting with embracing new challenges.*

◆ If you chose mostly Bs, you welcome a growth mindset. *Consider maintaining a resilient attitude of persevering in the face of adversity.*

◆ If you chose mostly Cs, you're leaning toward a growth mindset. *Continue to work on embracing failure as an opportunity for growth.*

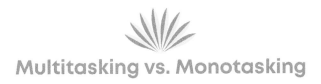

Multitasking vs. Monotasking

Our time is an incredibly valuable asset. While multitasking might make us feel productive in the moment, according to a 2001 research study, we're likely less efficient than we think. This is because it takes time to quickly switch between various tasks, so instead of doing multiple things simultaneously, we're actually rapidly shifting our focus between different activities.

The next time you're tempted to multitask, try monotasking, or single-tasking, instead. Commit yourself to one task with minimal distractions, and set a timer to help with time management. As monotasking can require more sustained focus than multitasking, set yourself up for success by first identifying what period of the day you tend to be most focused and productive.

Monotasking might promote an increased sense of mindfulness as you focus your efforts on one thing at a time and do each thing well. Reexamine your perception of productivity as you experiment with being more intentional and present in your pursuits.

The voice of your inner critic may not be your own. It may belong to someone you cared about and felt criticized by as a child (a parent, caregiver, sibling, etc.). Reflect on whose voice your self-critical thoughts may be taking on.

Disrupt the Cycle of Overthinking

Overthinking is the act of thinking or worrying about something excessively, sometimes to the point of mental exhaustion.
While overthinking can be confused with problem-solving, in reality, it offers a false sense of control and creates a cycle of anxiety and rumination.

Describe how you know when you're overthinking.

....

....

....

List some facts about the situation (not your thoughts or emotions).

....

....

....

Reframe your anxious thought with a positive perspective.

....

....

....

Replace your worry with a comforting thought.

....

....

....

Practice self-compassion by creating a self-affirmation or listing your strengths.

....

....

....

Noticing when you're overthinking is the first step to disrupting circular thinking. Once you've noticed anxious thoughts, you can find peace by reframing and replacing these thoughts with self-compassion.

Self-sabotage describes behavior that hinders progress toward your goals despite your desire to achieve them. How have you self-sabotaged in the past (procrastination, substance misuse, stress eating, etc.)? Why do you think you did so (fear, anxiety, insecurity, etc.)?

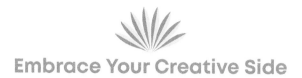

Embrace Your Creative Side

According to a 2016 study published in *The Journal of Positive Psychology*, tapping into creativity can increase your positive affect—your capacity to experience emotions such as happiness, optimism, and joy.

Creative expression through music, visual arts, dance, and writing has been found to reduce symptoms of depression and decrease stress levels. Research shows that creative experiences can have a protective effect on the brain, as engaging in artistic activities (such as painting, drawing, woodworking, etc.) in middle and old age might postpone cognitive decline.

You don't have to be an art prodigy to enjoy the creativity that lives within you! Here are some ideas for creative expression:

- Learn a new craft.
- Design an exercise routine.
- Create a photo collage.
- Plant a garden (indoors or out!).
- Doodle or color.
- Write a song.
- Choreograph a dance.
- Try a new recipe.

Challenge yourself to incorporate creativity into your daily life. Notice the impact that creativity can have on how you perceive yourself, others, and the world around you.

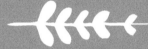

My thoughts are just thoughts. I watch them
float through my mind without judging them
or allowing them to define me.

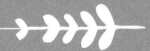

Identify something in your life that you've been struggling with. Write a compassionate and encouraging letter to yourself to help you cope with this challenge. If this feels difficult, write to yourself with the voice you'd use when speaking to a dear friend.

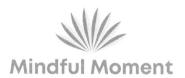

Mindful Moment

Mindfulness practices can help you mentally recenter yourself and feel more at ease. Engage in this meditation for as long as you'd like. Set a timer if you need to.

1. Find a comfortable position. Close your eyes or lower your gaze to minimize distractions.

2. Listen closely to the sounds around you, and identify as many as you can.

3. Now shift your focus to your body, noting the sensation of gravity pulling it down and creating a calming sense of heaviness.

4. Bring your attention to your breath, observing it as it enters your body, fills your lungs, and leaves your body. Take your time as you become in tune with your breathing.

5. When your mind wanders, simply acknowledge your thought and gently bring your focus back to your breath.

6. Gradually shift your awareness back to the sensation of your body, and then to the sounds around you.

7. Whenever you're ready, slowly wake up your body by wiggling your fingers and toes and opening your eyes.

Reflect on your experience with this mindfulness practice. What sensations did you feel in your body? What thoughts or emotions came up for you?

List five things that paint a picture of how you'd like your life to look in two years.

1. ....

2. ....

3. ....

4. ....

5. ....

Now list five ways you'd like your life to feel in two years, regardless of how it looks.

1. ....

2. ....

3. ....

4. ....

5. ....

Do you procrastinate? If so, it's time to confront your procrastination head-on and regain control over it. Though this might feel uncomfortable, be honest with yourself in listing five specific things you've been avoiding lately that need your attention (tasks, deadlines, relationships, personal goals, etc.).

1. ....

....

2. ....

....

3. ....

....

4. ....

....

5. ....

....

Control

What's your relationship with control? Check True or False, answering each question honestly without judging yourself for your response. Then, reflect on your answers.

	True	False
I find myself micromanaging situations often.		
I'd rather complete a task on my own than with others.		
My way of doing things is typically the best.		
I rarely delegate tasks to other people.		
I rarely let things naturally run their course.		
It's difficult for me to accept uncertainty.		
I strive for perfection.		
I criticize myself for making mistakes.		
It's hard for me to accept help from others.		
I struggle when things don't go according to my schedule.		
I feel very stressed when things don't go my way.		
Reality typically doesn't live up to my expectations.		
I tend to judge people who are different from me.		

Count up all the "True" responses:

9 or more: You likely struggle with control. Consider whether your need for control is negatively impacting your mental health and/or relationships.

4 to 8: You might struggle with control, but you are making progress in loosening your grip.

0 to 3: You're comfortable with not always being in control and welcome life as it unfolds.

Remember, there's nothing inherently wrong with knowing what you want and striving to be in control of your life. However, the desire to control can be problematic when it begins to negatively impact your mental health and relationships. Be patient with yourself as you learn to let go and embrace your life as it naturally unfolds.

It's natural to turn to unhealthy behaviors as a way to cope with stress. What potentially harmful coping skill can you reexamine your relationship with to improve your health? Examples include alcohol and substance use, disordered eating, and excessive spending.

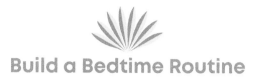

Build a Bedtime Routine

Mental health and sleep are intertwined. Research has shown that sleep impacts brain health by facilitating improved cognition, learning, and memory. Also, according to the National Heart, Lung, and Blood Institute, restful sleep helps the brain and body recover during the night, while conversely, sleep deprivation can increase the risk for physical health problems such as heart disease, high blood pressure, diabetes, and more.

Good sleep hygiene involves cultivating daily routines that help you achieve consistent, uninterrupted, and restful sleep. Use the following guide to help build your bedtime routine and nurture your mental and physical health:

◆ Choose your bedtime and wake-up time and stick to them.

◆ Schedule 20 to 30 minutes for winding down before you sleep.

◆ Turn off all screens 30 to 60 minutes before bedtime.

◆ Maintain a comfortable temperature in your bedroom.

◆ Use relaxation techniques such as meditation, stretching, and deep breathing.

◆ Avoid caffeine, alcohol, or big meals close to your bedtime.

◆ Journal your thoughts and experiences from the day.

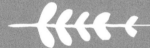

I accept that there are things out of my control. I welcome uncertainty with curiosity, confidence, and optimism.

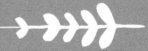

Failure is a natural part of growth and can offer valuable information about which approaches to your goals are working and which are not working. What's something that you feel you've failed at? How can you embrace this failure, and what can you learn from it?

_____

_____

_____

_____

_____

_____

_____

_____

_____

_____

_____

_____

Identify a belief you have about yourself that holds you back. When did it first begin? What is it rooted in (past experiences, comments from others, etc.)? Explore how this self-limiting belief has impacted you in the past and present.

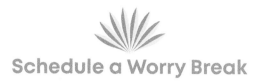

Schedule a Worry Break

Anxiety can feed a vicious cycle of stress and overthinking. Set aside time for a daily worry break! This can help you manage your anxiety, release stress, and find peace.

◆ Schedule 10 to 15 minutes a day to focus on what's been worrying you.

◆ Commit to taking your worry deep dive around the same time each day.

◆ If you notice yourself worrying during the day, write down your thoughts to revisit during your next deep dive.

◆ It might be helpful to organize your anxious thoughts into two categories: "things I can control" and "things I can't control."

◆ During your worry break, examine your anxiety. Ask yourself questions like, "What would I like to happen?" and "What can I do first?"

◆ When your worry deep dive is over, refocus your energy on a new task. If you feel fixated on anxious thoughts, remember that you can come back to them during your next worry break. Write them down to revisit later.

Use this space to release your anxious thoughts during your worry deep dive. This is an opportunity to finally set down the stress you've been carrying.

Personalization is a common thinking trap in which we wrongfully assume responsibility for negative outcomes that were, in actuality, out of our control. What are some things you've blamed yourself for that you now realize were not in your complete control?

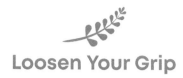

Loosen Your Grip

Having a moderate sense of control in our life can help us feel safe and secure. However, the desire or need to excessively control things can negatively impact our mental health and show up in ways such as overthinking, overplanning, and doubting ourselves and others. A need for control is often rooted in the fear that something will go wrong. Reflect on one thing you've been trying to excessively control, then give yourself the reassurance you deserve by filling in the blanks. Repeat this statement out loud whenever you feel the need to.

Today, I loosen my grip on trying to control _____

(situation/event). I release my anxiety and welcome peace into

my life. If I find myself worrying about this, I'll _____

(healthy coping skill) or reach out to _____ (social

support) for support. I've coped with every unplanned situation

in my life so far, and I know that things will work out, even if not

exactly the way I planned. Today, I choose to trust myself and

the process.

Many of us minimize the good and magnify the bad in our lives. This can negatively impact our mental health over time. List five good things in your life that you've been minimizing lately, no matter how big or small.

1. ....

....

2. ....

....

3. ....

....

4. ....

....

5. ....

....

It can be easy to internalize negative thoughts. Unfortunately, they can cause our mental health to deteriorate. What are some anxious, uncomfortable, or unhelpful thoughts that you've been having? Put some distance between yourself and your thoughts, and remind yourself that they're just thoughts.

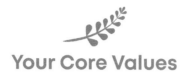

Your Core Values

Values "are the principles that give our lives meaning and allow us to persevere through adversity," according to psychologist Barb Markway and writer Celia Ampel. Your values can serve as anchors and remind you of what truly matters to you.

Here, you'll consider your **core values**, or the principles that are most important to you. If this feels difficult, consider the traits of people whom you admire. Circle up to seven core values, writing in additional values if they aren't already listed.

Acceptance	Balance	Diversity	Health	Creativity
Family	Compassion	Love	Faith	Playfulness
Humility	Justice	Independence	Gratitude	Leadership
Discipline	Optimism	Education	Adventure	Harmony
Privacy	Cleanliness	Pleasure	Knowledge	Vulnerability
Respect	Security	Humor	Kindness	Community
Spirituality	Trust	Loyalty	Beauty	Courage
Collaboration	Integrity	Openness	Empathy	Passion
Flexibility	Confidence	Resilience	Consistency	Helpfulness

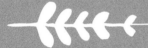

I will pursue my goals no matter what obstacles I face. I know I am worthy of achieving them.

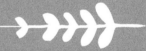

Part
Three

Thrive in Your Social Life

Research has shown that people with strong and supportive relationships tend to live longer, healthier lives and are less likely to experience anxiety and depression. It doesn't matter how many friends you have or whether you have a romantic partner. Rather, it's the *quality* of your relationships that impacts your mental health.

Part three of this journal will help you reflect on your past experiences in relationships, gain helpful communication tools, and identify barriers to experiencing more fulfilling and meaningful relationships. Some topics you'll explore include self-trust, boundaries, forgiveness, effective communication, compassion, and more.

You'll be guided through exercises to help you examine your identity and practice self-care so you can show up as your best self for yourself and others. As you engage in this intimate inner work, take the time to acknowledge uncomfortable emotions or memories if they arise, and honor your limits. As you progress through this section, challenge yourself to stretch to new places, and don't forget to enjoy the process of getting to know yourself better. After all, our relationship with ourselves sets the tone for our relationships with others.

Identify one relationship in your life that is lacking healthy boundaries. How can you set boundaries with this person to protect your mental and emotional well-being? Ideally, how would your relationship with this person change compared to how it is now?

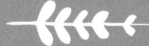

I deserve to feel respected and appreciated in my relationships and to surround
myself with people who bring me joy.

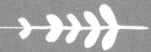

How Healthy Are Your Boundaries?

Choose the response that best describes your comfort with setting boundaries with others. Remember, there are no wrong answers.

1. When I'm asked a question I don't want to answer . . .
   A. I answer it anyway.
   B. I don't answer it, but feel guilty.
   C. I'm comfortable not answering it.

2. When I'm asked to do something that I don't have time for . . .
   A. I struggle to say "no."
   B. I reluctantly end up doing it.
   C. I don't agree to it.

3. When someone hurts me . . .
   A. I pretend I'm unbothered.
   B. I act passive-aggressively.
   C. I let them know how I feel.

Insights

◆ If you chose mostly As, setting boundaries with others might be challenging. *Try remembering that healthy relationships have boundaries.*

◆ If you chose mostly Bs, your boundaries with others can be strengthened. *Consider experimenting with expressing your emotions more directly.*

◆ If you chose mostly Cs, you're comfortable setting boundaries with others. *Continue to honor your needs and nurture your mental health.*

Consider your comfort levels in various social situations (meeting new people, talking on the phone, eating in front of others, etc.). What social situations make you feel the most comfortable? Which ones make you feel less comfortable, perhaps even anxious?

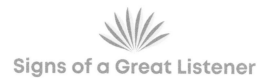

Signs of a Great Listener

Good listening is essential for good communication. To gauge whether your active listening skills are at their best, reflect on these five tips:

1. **Be present.** If your mind becomes distracted, gently acknowledge your distracted thoughts and bring your attention back to the conversation.

2. **Listen to understand, not to respond.** Instead of focusing on what you'll say, focus on processing what's being shared with you.

3. **Resist the urge to interrupt.** It can make the other person feel dismissed, so save your questions and comments until they're finished speaking.

4. **Ask follow-up questions.** After you've processed what they've shared, ask questions that elicit more detailed information.

5. **Show that you're listening.** Use active body language such as eye contact, an alert expression, or an encouraging nod of your head.

Being an intentional listener helps build strong relationships and allows us to practice mindfulness. People enjoy speaking with good listeners because they feel genuinely heard and understood.

What are three strengths you bring to your relationships? What are three things you'd like to work on in yourself to improve your relationships? As you reflect, keep in mind that no personal strength or area of growth is too small.

Strengths

1. ....

....

2. ....

....

3. ....

....

Things I Can Improve

1. ....

....

2. ....

....

3. ....

....

An Impactful Relationship

Whether with caregivers, friends, romantic partners, peers, or someone else, both nurturing *and* harmful interactions with others have the capacity to shape us.

Identify one relationship that has significantly shaped you:

My relationship with ....

....

List three ways this person has influenced how you see yourself:

1. ....

2. ....

3. ....

How has this person impacted how you treat other people and function in your relationships?

....

....

....

....

What are three valuable lessons that you've learned from this relationship?

1. ....

2. ....

3. ....

Reflect on whether there's anything you've learned in your relationship with this person that you'd like to *unlearn*. Acknowledging this does not minimize positive aspects of your relationship with them.

....

....

....

What's one thing you'd like this person to know?

....

....

....

Remember this: Regardless of how your relationships have shaped *you*, you are your own person. *You* get to decide what kind of person you want to be and what impact you'd like to have in this world.

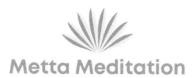

Metta Meditation

Metta meditation, also known as "loving-kindness meditation," is a traditional Buddhist practice that involves repeating kind phrases to yourself and others.

1. Find a comfortable position, and close your eyes or lower your gaze to minimize distractions. Take several slow, deep breaths.

2. Begin by opening your heart to your own well-being. Silently repeat the following phrases:

   May I be happy.
   May I be healthy.
   May I be at ease.

3. Now think of someone you care about. Silently offer this person the same phrases of loving-kindness:

   May you be happy.
   May you be healthy.
   May you be at ease.

4. Next, think of someone whom you find difficult, annoying, or draining and offer them the same phrases of loving-kindness. Recognize that, just like you, this person wants to feel happy, healthy, safe, and at ease.

5. Repeat this practice with others in mind, such as neighbors, acquaintances, and animals.

6. Shift your attention to your breathing. Whenever you're ready, slowly open your eyes.

How do you feel after completing this metta meditation? What thoughts and emotions came up for you as you offered phrases of loving-kindness to others in your life?

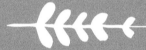

I'm not for everyone, and everyone's not for me. I relinquish the need to please or be liked by everyone.

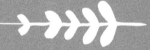

Our identity is influenced by our relationships with others. List five of your social roles or titles that you value the most (sister, friend, employee, etc.). Beside each one, write a note about how this role has shaped you.

1. ....

....

2. ....

....

3. ....

....

4. ....

....

5. ....

....

Self-Boundary Check-In

How well do you honor your personal boundaries? Check True, False, or Unsure, without judging yourself for your responses. Then, view your insights.

	True	False	Unsure
I prioritize time for myself.			
I don't contact people who are meant to stay in my past.			
I honor my needs.			
I allow myself to rest when I feel tired.			
I advocate for myself.			
I make decisions that align with my values.			
I hold myself accountable for my actions.			
I feel comfortable saying "no" to people.			
I seek out support when I need it.			
I stick to my budget.			
I don't engage in things that are unhealthy for me.			

Insights

◆ Any "True" responses indicate strengths with honoring your personal boundaries.

◆ Any "False" and "Unsure" responses may indicate areas of opportunity to set healthier boundaries with yourself.

Our relationship with ourselves sets the tone for every other relationship in our life.

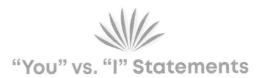

"You" vs. "I" Statements

"I" statements highlight your thoughts and feelings while "you" statements focus on another person's behavior. "You" statements tend to take on an accusatory tone. It's important to know that "I" statements do not minimize or condone other people's hurtful behaviors; rather, they can help you express your emotions and facilitate productive communication.

Pioneering psychologist Dr. Thomas Gordon describes three main elements of "I" statements:

- The behavior that upset you

- How it makes you feel

- How it affects you

View the following example of an "I" statement:

"YOU" Statement	"I" Statement
You never listen to me.	**I** feel hurt [feelings] when you constantly interrupt me [behavior], because it makes it difficult for me to fully express myself [effect].

Try using "I" statements the next time you wish to address a conflict with someone.

Expressing your emotions and acknowledging the impact that someone has on you takes courage and vulnerability. If expressing yourself in this way feels foreign, remember that it will get easier with practice.

Identify five qualities that you value most in your relationships with other people (trust, respect, honesty, etc.). Consider relationships of all kinds, such as those with family, friends, peers, or romantic partners. What makes these qualities so important to you?

Perception

In the inner circle, write words that describe how you see yourself. In the outer circle, write words that you think others would use to describe you. If it's challenging to completely separate your self-perception from others' perceptions of you, that's okay. The two are often intertwined.

What similarities and differences do you notice about how you perceive yourself and how others perceive you?

....

....

....

What are five words that describe the real you? Take a moment to appreciate yourself just as you are today:

1. ....

2. ....

3. ....

4. ....

5. ....

What are three things that you'd like others (friends, family members, colleagues, romantic partners, etc.) to know about you?

1. ....

2. ....

3. ....

You deserve to feel appreciated for who you authentically are, by others and yourself.

How well can you trust yourself? When do you trust yourself the most, and when is it more difficult to tap into your instincts? Reflect on your confidence with decision-making, and consider how important receiving validation from others is to you.

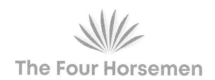

The Four Horsemen

Researcher and relationship expert Dr. John Gottman uncovered four negative behaviors, which he calls "the four horsemen," that can contribute to the end of a relationship. Reflect on what people or situations might trigger the four horsemen in your communication with others.

When you are tempted to use the four horsemen in your relationships, counter them by using their antidotes instead.

Four Horsemen	Antidotes
Criticism: Attacking someone's character (e.g., "You never think about my emotions") instead of offering constructive feedback	Start gently ◆ Focus on the problem, not the person. ◆ Use "I" statements.
Contempt: Treating someone disrespectfully by mocking them, or using dismissive body language like eye-rolling	Practice compassion ◆ Recognize their strengths. ◆ Acknowledge their efforts.
Defensiveness: Protecting yourself from criticism by blaming others and taking no personal responsibility	Take responsibility ◆ Consider their perspective. ◆ Apologize for any harm you may have caused.
Stonewalling: Disengaging and shutting down to avoid conflict instead of confronting the problem	Self-soothe ◆ Use relaxation techniques (e.g., deep breathing). ◆ Pause the conversation.

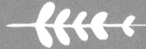

I love myself just as I am. The more I love myself, the more I love my relationships with others.

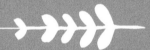

Who are the people in your life that energize you?
Conversely, who are the people that drain your energy?
What is it about these relationships that makes
them feel either rejuvenating or tiring?

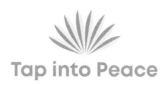

Tap into Peace

1. Sit back or lie down in a comfortable position, and close your eyes if you're comfortable doing so.

2. Take several slow, deep breaths. Picture your body becoming oxygenated and replenished with each long inhale and stress leaving your body with each long exhale.

3. Visualize a majestic, beautiful mountain that reaches into the clouds. Allow the image to gradually come into focus. Perhaps your mountain has high peaks or snowcapped tops. Maybe it's lush with rivers, trees, and meadows.

4. Imagine what you hear, such as chirping birds or a babbling brook. Consider what you smell, such as fresh pine or crisp, clean air. Envision what you feel, such as cool air in your nostrils or rough bark on a tree.

5. Become one with the mountain in your mind's eye. Like the mountain, you are majestic, peaceful, and grounded.

6. Allow yourself to get lost in this visualization. Continue breathing deeply and conclude this practice whenever you feel ready.

How do you feel after visualizing and experiencing the mountain you created? Notice how you feel now in comparison to how you felt before this visualization.

What are three important lessons you've learned from previous relationships? Reflect on past relationships of all kinds, such as those with family, friends, or romantic partners. How can they guide and improve your present and future relationships?

1.

2.

3.

List three things you'd like to share with someone you care about. Perhaps what you wish to share is lighthearted, or maybe it's more serious and has been on your mind for a while. Communication is key to healthy relationships.

1. ....

....

....

2. ....

....

....

3. ....

....

....

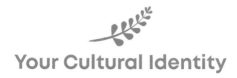

Your Cultural Identity

Culture can describe the shared knowledge, values, and practices of a group of people, whether it's a family, community, ethnic group, etc. Culture can also describe ways of life that encompass language, social norms, religion, art, food, music, and more.

Whether your culture is one that you were born into, adopted later on, or have modified over time, reflect on how it has shaped your social identity and worldview:

I describe my ethnic and cultural background as:

....

....

Three words that describe people in my cultural group are:

1. ....

2. ....

3. ....

Three things I appreciate about my culture are:

1. ....

2. ....

3. ....

Three things I've outgrown from my culture are:

1. ....

2. ....

3. ....

Something I wish people understood about my culture is:

....

....

....

My culture impacts the way I view my relationships by:

....

....

....

Three cultural or family traditions I want to share with others are:

1. ....

2. ....

3. ....

What's your deepest fear when it comes to relationships? How has this fear held you back from feeling authentic and secure in your relationships? Put this fear into words, and experience the freedom that comes with letting it out.

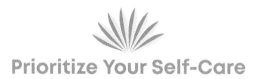

Prioritize Your Self-Care

Self-care has a multitude of physical and mental benefits. How can you incorporate simple self-care practices into your daily routine? Brainstorm, using the following ideas for inspiration if you feel stuck.

Give myself a compliment.	Spend time in nature.	Meal prep for tomorrow.	Take a nap.
Stretch my body.	Go for a walk.	Listen to relaxing music.	Create a skincare routine.
Drink some water.	Take a warm bath.	Make my bed.	Craft or doodle.
Dance to my favorite song.	Journal my thoughts.	Wash the dishes.	Identify my values.
Go to sleep earlier than usual.	Unplug from technology.	Make a budget for the month.	Try something new.
Organize my space.	Declutter my inbox.	Meditate for three minutes.	Watch a funny video.
Read a good book.	Reach out to a friend.	Nourish my body.	Finish a task on my to-do list.

At the end of the day, acknowledge what you accomplished and forgive yourself for what you didn't get to. Remember that tomorrow brings new opportunities.

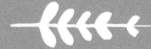

I set healthy boundaries in my relationships.
I respect the emotions of others as well
as my own.

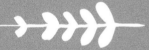

Write a letter to someone you feel ready to forgive. Forgiveness doesn't mean that what happened was okay. Rather, it means you feel ready to experience freedom from the pain you endured. Don't do it for them; do it for yourself.

Growth is often accompanied by discomfort and sometimes even pain. What behaviors, relationships, or people have you outgrown over the course of your life? What people or things were particularly difficult to leave behind once you realized that you'd outgrown them?

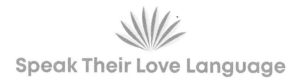

Speak Their Love Language

According to author Dr. Gary Chapman, there are five main love languages that people tend to respond to.

Identify a loved one with whom you'd like to strengthen your relationship. Perhaps it's a friend, family member, or romantic partner. Consider what their primary love language is, and follow through with a related action to express your affection.

Love Language	Ideas for Actions to Take
Words of affirmation	Communicate praise, appreciation, empathy, and encouragement.
Physical touch	Hold hands, hug, offer a massage, or cuddle with them.
Receiving gifts	Present them with a thoughtful gift, no matter how small or inexpensive.
Quality time	Offer your undivided attention, make eye contact, and actively listen to them.
Acts of service	Help them tackle their to-do list, and prioritize their needs and wants.

Recognizing other people's love languages can help you express affection in the ways they most appreciate and allow you to connect on a deeper level.

How did it feel offering affection to this person in accordance with their love language? How did they respond? Reflect on what makes this person so important to you.

What does love mean to you? Does love look different across different kinds of relationships (platonic, familial, romantic, etc.) in your life? If you haven't experienced love yet, write about how you imagine it will feel when it happens.

Are You a People Pleaser?

There is nothing inherently wrong with wanting to please others. However, if you prioritize others' happiness at the expense of your own, it can take a toll on your mental health.

Check True or False for each prompt below, and then view your insights.

	True	False
I often seek validation from others.		
I avoid confrontation with others at all costs.		
I feel responsible for other people's emotions.		
I strive to be liked by everyone.		
I tend to over-apologize.		
My self-worth depends on what others think.		
I feel guilty putting myself first.		
I struggle with asserting my needs.		

Count up all the "True" responses:

6 or more: This is a good time to consider whether people pleasing is negatively impacting your mental and emotional well-being.

3 to 5: You sacrifice a lot for others, but you are working on asserting yourself more.

0 to 2: You acknowledge your needs and are comfortable setting boundaries with others.

Identify five people you care about, including yourself. For each person, consider one way you can express support in a manner that they'd appreciate. Consider their personal preferences and what would be the most meaningful to them. Remember to do this for yourself, too!

1. ....

....

2. ....

....

3. ....

....

4. ....

....

5. ....

....

How comfortable are you with confronting others and handling conflict in your relationships? Does your comfort vary based on the relationship? Reflect on your conflict resolution style, how effective it's been in the past, and whether you'd like to do anything differently going forward.

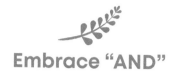

Embrace "AND"

As we explored in part 1, a dialectical statement acknowledges two opposing yet simultaneous truths. Create space for the duality of your emotions as you reflect on the past, make peace with the present, and embrace the future.

I can forgive

_____   *AND*   still choose not to let
(someone who hurt you badly   them back into my life at
that you purposely don't   this time.
speak to)

I can grieve the loss of

_____   *AND*   still feel hopeful for good
(someone or something that   things to enter my life.
still weighs heavily on your
heart)

I can deeply care about

_____   *AND*   still set healthy boundar-
(someone who's special to   ies with them.
you)

I can move on from

_____   *AND*   still think about it
(a painful experience that   sometimes.
you've healed from)

Hold space for the complexity of your emotions and experiences.

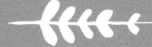

I compassionately hold space for other people's emotions without internalizing them as my own.

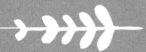

Resources

Here are some books to further your exploration of the mind-brain interaction, mental and emotional wellness, healthy relationships, and more:

Attached: The New Science of Adult Attachment and How It Can Help You Find—and Keep—Love by Dr. Amir Levine and Rachel S. F. Heller, MA

The 5 Love Languages: The Secret to Love That Lasts by Gary Chapman

Happiness by Design: Change What You Do, Not How You Think by Paul Dolan, PhD

Incognito: The Secret Lives of the Brain by David Eagleman

It Didn't Start with You: How Inherited Family Trauma Shapes Who We Are and How to End the Cycle by Mark Wolynn

Milk and Honey by Rupi Kaur

Thriving as an Empath: 365 Days of Self-Care for Sensitive People by Judith Orloff, MD

52-Week Mental Health Journal: Guided Prompts and Self-Reflection to Reduce Stress and Improve Wellbeing by Cynthia Catchings, LCSW-S, LCSW-C, MSSW

The CBT Workbook for Mental Health: Evidence-Based Exercises to Transform Negative Thoughts and Manage Your Well-Being by Simon A. Rego, PsyD and Sarah Fader

Self-Love Workbook for Women: Release Self-Doubt, Build Self-Compassion, and Embrace Who You Are by Megan Logan, MSW, LCSW

References

Adams, Michelle. "What are the Essential Components of an I-Message?" Gordon Training International. May 31, 2012. www.gordontraining.com/leadership/what-are-the-essential -components-of-an-i-message.

Conner, Tamlin S., Colin G. DeYoung, and Paul J. Silvia. "Everyday Creative Activity as a Path to Flourishing." *The Journal of Positive Psychology.* 13, no. 2 (November 2016): 181–189. doi.org /10.1080/17439760.2016.1257049.

Doran, George. "There's a S.M.A.R.T. Way to Write Management's Goals and Objectives." *Management Review* 70, no. 11 (November 1981): 35-36.

Gottlieb, Andrea Lee Barrocas. "DBT 101: What Does 'Dialectical' Even Mean?" Sheppard Pratt. October 26, 2016. www .sheppardpratt.org/news-views/story/dbt-101-what-does -dialectical-even-mean.

The Gottman Institute. "4 Conflict Styles That Hurt Your Relationship." January 25, 2021. www.gottman.com/blog/4-conflict -styles-that-hurt-your-relationship.

Holt-Lunstad, Julianne, Timothy Smith, and J. Bradley Layton. "Social Relationships and Mortality Risk: A Meta-analytic Review." *PLOS Medicine* 7, no. 7 (July 2010): e1000316. doi.org/10.1371/journal.pmed.1000316.

Lisitsa, Ellie. "The Four Horsemen: The Antidotes." The Gottman Institute. April 26, 2013. www.gottman.com/blog/the-four -horsemen-the-antidotes.

Maquet, Pierre. "Sleep On It!" *Nature Neuroscience* 3, no. 12 (December 2000): 1235–1236. doi.org/10.1038/81750.

Markway, Barbara and Celia Ampel. *The Self-Confidence Workbook: A Guide to Overcoming Self-Doubt and Improving Self-Esteem.* Emeryville, CA: Althea Press, 2018.

National Heart, Lung, and Blood Institute. "Sleep Deprivation and Deficiency." Accessed on August 17, 2021. www.nhlbi .nih.gov/health-topics/sleep-deprivation-and-deficiency.

National Institute of Mental Health. "Women and Mental Health." Last modified May 2019. www.nimh.nih.gov/health/topics /women-and-mental-health.

Nunez, Kirsten. "5 Benefits of Metta Meditation and How to Do It." Healthline. June 9, 2020. www.healthline.com/health /metta-meditation.

Roberts, Rosebud O., Ruth H. Cha, Michelle M. Mielke, Yonas E. Geda, Bradley F. Boeve, Mary M. Machulda, David S. Knopman, and Ronald C. Petersen. "Risk and Protective Factors for Cognitive Impairment in Persons Aged 85 Years and Older." *Neurology* 84, no. 18 (May 2015): 1854–1861. doi.org/10.1212 /WNL.0000000000001537.

Rubinstein, Joshua S., David E. Meyer, and Jeffrey E. Evans. "Executive Control of Cognitive Processes in Task Switching." *Journal of Experimental Psychology: Human Perception and Performance* 27, no. 4 (January 2001): 763–797. doi.org/10.1037 /0096-1523.27.4.763.

Santini, Ziggi Ivan, Ai Koyanagi, Stefanos Tyrovolas, and Josep M. Haro. "The Association of Relationship Quality and Social Networks with Depression, Anxiety, and Suicidal Ideation among Older Married Adults: Findings from a Cross-Sectional Analysis of the Irish Longitudinal Study on Ageing (TILDA)." *Journal of*

Affective Disorders 179 (July 2015): 134–141. doi.org/10.1016
/j.jad.2015.03.015.

Saxbe, Darby and Rena Repetti. "No Place Like Home: Home
Tours Correlate with Daily Patterns of Mood and Cortisol."
Personality and Social Psychology Bulletin 36, no. 1 (January
2010): 71–81. doi.org/10.1177/0146167209352864.

Stuckey, Heather L. and Jeremy Nobel. "The Connection Between
Art, Healing, and Public Health: A Review of Current Litera-
ture." *American Journal of Public Health* 100, no. 2 (May 2009):
254–263. doi.org/10.2105/AJPH.2008.156497.

Teo, Alan R., Hwajung Choi, and Marcia Valenstein. "Social
Relationships and Depression: Ten-Year Follow-Up from a
Nationally Representative Study." *PLOS One* 8, no. 4 (April
2013). doi.org/10.1371/journal.pone.0062396.

Tolin, David F. *Doing CBT: A Comprehensive Guide to Working
with Behaviors, Thoughts, and Emotions.* New York, NY: The
Guilford Press, 2016.

Acknowledgments

Curtis, my devoted husband, thank you for inspiring me to always believe in myself and my capabilities. Mom and Dad, you have always been my biggest fans, and I have endless gratitude for your steadfast support in my life. Samira, my sister and best friend, thank you for always inspiring me to be my authentic self. Nani, Nana, Achie, and Thatha, thank you for guiding me with the love of Jesus Christ. I love you all very much!

About the Author

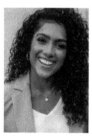 **Sana Isaac Powell, MA, LPC,** is a holistic and culturally affirming licensed professional counselor, advocate, and educator. Her desire to make mental health resources more inclusive is inspired by her clinical work with diverse populations as well as her personal experiences as a first-generation Indian-American woman. She enjoys writing about and demystifying mental health topics to help others lead healthier and happier lives. Her favorite forms of self-care include journaling, watching *The Great British Baking Show*, and hiking with her husband, Curtis, and canine companion, River. Find her on Instagram @curly_therapist and at SanaPowell.com.

CPSIA information can be obtained
at www.ICGtesting.com
Printed in the USA
JSHW012005240722
28021JS00001B/2

9 781638 788812